KATIE PRUITT

Healthy & Fit Moms

A guide for busy moms on losing weight and getting back in shape after babies

Contents

1

Overview of the book

"Healthy & Fit Moms: A guide for busy moms on losing weight and getting back in shape after babies" is a comprehensive and empowering resource tailored specifically for mothers who are navigating the challenges of postpartum life while striving to prioritize their health and fitness. Written with empathy and understanding, this book serves as a road map for busy moms looking to reclaim their bodies, boost their energy levels, and foster a renewed sense of confidence and vitality.

At its core, "Healthy & Fit Moms" recognizes the unique obstacles that mothers face when it comes to achieving their health and fitness goals. From the physical toll of pregnancy and childbirth to the demands of caring for young children, many moms find themselves overwhelmed and unsure of where to begin. This book seeks to provide guidance and support every step of the way, offering practical strategies and actionable advice that can be seamlessly integrated into even the busiest of schedules.

The book begins with the author's personal story where readers are introduced to a real-life mom who has successfully implemented intermittent fasting and exercise into her routine, inspiring hope and confidence in their own abilities to achieve similar results. Then the book outlines the importance of self-care for moms and provides a brief history of intermittent fasting—a key component of the program in the book.

From there, "Healthy & Fit Moms" delves into the nuts and bolts of intermittent fasting, explaining the science behind this powerful eating pattern and detailing its numerous health benefits. Readers will learn about different approaches to intermittent fasting and how to customize their fasting schedule to suit their individual preferences and lifestyle.

But "Healthy & Fit Moms" goes beyond just intermittent fasting, recognizing the importance of incorporating regular exercise into a healthy lifestyle. Readers will discover practical tips for finding the time and motivation to exercise, as well as guidance on choosing activities that are enjoyable and sustainable.

Throughout the book, readers will find helpful strategies for overcoming common challenges and staying consistent on their health and fitness journey. From dealing with hunger pangs during fasting periods to managing time constraints and finding support from loved ones, "Healthy & Fit Moms" provides the tools and encouragement needed to overcome obstacles and stay on track towards achieving their goals.

In the end, "Healthy & Fit Moms" is more than just a book—it's a lifeline for mothers who are ready to prioritize their health and well-being, reclaim their bodies, and embrace the transformative power of self-care. With its practical advice, inspiring stories, and unwavering support, this book is sure to empower and uplift busy moms everywhere as they embark on their own journey to becoming healthy, fit, and thriving.

2

My Story

Allow me to introduce myself. My name is Katie and I am wife to Justin and mommy to Abner, Sebastian, Jacob, and Rosalie–all 6 years and under. Sound a bit crazy already? Believe me, it is. But we have fun!

I've never been one who was naturally thin. I've always had to be very conscious of what I ate and work at it. But I've always enjoyed health–eating healthy, exercising, doing things that feed my soul and fill me with joy. These things have always been easy to incorporate into my schedule…until I had kids. Hello world turned upside down! It has never been a bad thing, I wanted children and I love being a mom! But it has most definitely been a very challenging thing. My first two babies, Abner and Sebastian, are twins. It was so much fun getting that news! My husband and I laughed the whole way home. I wanted twins. I prayed for twins! I got twins. (insert blissful face)

Man, did that pregnancy do a number on my body. As I said, I'm not naturally thin by any means. In fact, if I let it, my body would happily gain a million pounds easily. When I became pregnant with the twins, I got morning sickness pretty intensely. It calmed down a few months in, but I had food aversions the entire pregnancy. The way I used to eat, all healthy and so many salads and hardly any bread and rarely any fried foods or junk—all that went out the window. I ate whatever I could stomach or whatever I was craving. I *tried* to stay healthy with my eating, somewhat, but it was very difficult with the way I was feeling so much of the time. Here's what I'm getting at: I gained 80 pounds with that pregnancy by the end. You read me right. I realize not all that was fat gained. My babies were just over six and a half pounds each! And I bloated so much in the last two months. After birth and a few weeks to let swelling and bloating go down, I still had somewhere around 30 pounds to lose. And those pounds were largely due to fat gained during pregnancy.

How did I lose it? At first it was just my attempts to go back to eating healthy. I was also breastfeeding, and they say that is supposed to help you lose weight. In my personal experience, I feel like breastfeeding makes losing weight difficult and slows it way down. It was like my body just wanted to hold on to the weight for dear life in order to have enough stored up to feed the babies. It was like this for each pregnancy!

I also managed to fit exercise into my day. Exercise to me is essential to not only my body's health, but also my mental and emotional health. It's a *must*! It was definitely more of a challenge now that I had two babies to look after. But I made it happen. I got a twin stroller and I took them on walks, just weeks old. When Justin was home, I got him to watch the twins while I took 30-45 minutes to do a workout video in our living room. On Justin's days off, we often would go off to the mountains for the day and go hiking, each carrying a baby.

Slowly, so slowly, but surely, the weight was coming off. I had gotten close to losing most of those pesky extra pounds when I discovered my secret weapon to losing weight, and it didn't require depriving myself of so many different foods that I love. Intermittent fasting! So many attempts to lose weight in the past have been with fad diets like the Paleo diet or the Keto diet or counting calories (I hate counting calories!).

Intermittent fasting was so much easier to implement and to sustain, and I lost weight faster!

When I was nearly back to my pre-baby weight, I got pregnant with Jacob. My body said, "Hey, I've done this before!" And the weight started coming right back on, more easily this time. Again, I was very sick, had food aversions, and ate whatever and whenever. By the end, I had gained 75 pounds and gave birth to a 10 pound 2 ounce baby (he's still huge!).

This time I had my secret weapon! Just a couple months postpartum I began implementing intermittent fasting and the pounds started melting away. So much easier. So much faster. I had hiccups along the way. Sometimes I didn't trust intermittent fasting and I went back to something else. Sometimes life happened, like holidays or birthday parties, and I got off intermittent fasting for a chunk of time. But always I kept coming back to it.

Exercise became even trickier to fit into my schedule, but I did it! Nap time is my favorite time. One of my biggest feats as a mother was when I got all three boys napping at the same time. Then it was me time! But sometimes, Jacob didn't nap at the same time the twins did. Then I'd just set him in his bouncy chair and he'd watch me as I worked out. Oftentimes, I'd take Jacob in the stroller and the twins would toddle along as we walked. Not the best workout, but still exercise! And I'm raising my boys to know and love exercise. And, of course, whenever Justin was around to help, I'd ask him to watch the babies so I could get a good workout in–by myself!

Then, when I was only a few pounds from the weight I started at before any babies, I got pregnant with Rosalie. I only gained 70 pounds this time (insert laughing face). After she was born, I jumped into intermittent fasting right off. This time around was the most difficult to get the weight off. But with intermittent fasting, trying to be mindful of eating healthy, and exercising in some way most days of the week, the weight has come off.

Was I able to lose all this postpartum weight (3 times!) easily? No, it was not easy. It took dedication, self-motivation, and hard work. Did it all just fall off naturally and without any kind of effort? Absolutely not. It took a lot of effort. Did it just all come off by itself because I'm just naturally thin? Heck no! As I've said already, my body loves to gain weight and does so *easily*. I have to be very mindful and diligent. And it took some time. The first 20 pounds came off within the first 5-6 months. The last 10 pounds took another 5-6 months. But I just kept trying, kept doing intermittent fasting, kept exercising, kept being mindful, and the pounds came off.

Losing weight and being fit is possible for *you* just as it is for me. And that's why I wrote this book. To explain how it is possible for you, amongst your crazy busy, mom-life schedule. Amongst all the pulls and tugs in the life of a busy mom, you too can be the *best* you. You *can* achieve your goals. You *can* lose weight. You *can* be fit. And I'll give you some tips and strategies to help you in your journey.

3

Importance of Self-Care for Moms

Self-care is crucial for busy moms, as it plays a fundamental role in maintaining physical, mental, and emotional well-being amidst the demands and responsibilities of motherhood. Here are several key reasons why self-care is essential for busy moms:

1. Physical Health: Taking care of one's physical health is essential for moms to have the energy and stamina needed to keep up with the demands of parenting. Self-care practices such as getting enough sleep, eating nutritious meals, staying hydrated, and engaging in regular exercise are vital for maintaining optimal physical health. Prioritizing self-care can help moms prevent burnout, reduce the risk of illness, and promote overall wellness.

2. Mental Health: The demands of motherhood can take a toll on mental health, leading to stress, anxiety, and feelings of being overwhelmed. Self-care practices such as mindfulness meditation, deep breathing exercises, journaling, and seeking therapy or counseling can help moms manage stress, improve mood, and cultivate a greater sense of emotional resilience. By prioritizing their mental health, moms can better cope with the challenges of

parenting and maintain a positive outlook on life.

3. Emotional Well-being: Self-care is essential for nurturing emotional well-being and fostering a sense of fulfillment and satisfaction in life. Moms often prioritize the needs of their families over their own, which can lead to feelings of neglect or resentment. Engaging in activities that bring joy, fulfillment, and a sense of purpose—whether it's pursuing a hobby, spending time with friends, or simply taking a moment to relax and unwind—can help moms recharge emotionally and maintain a healthy work-life balance.

4. Role Modeling: As parents, moms serve as powerful role models for their children, shaping their attitudes and behaviors towards self-care and wellness. By prioritizing their own self-care, moms demonstrate to their children the importance of taking care of oneself and setting healthy boundaries. Teaching children the value of self-care from a young age can help instill lifelong habits of self-love and self-respect.

5. Relationships: Prioritizing self-care can also strengthen relationships with partners, family members, and friends. When moms take the time to care for themselves, they are better able to show up fully present and engaged in their relationships, fostering deeper connections and intimacy. Additionally, self-care practices such as setting boundaries, communicating effectively, and practicing forgiveness can help moms navigate relationship challenges more effectively.

In essence, self-care is not a luxury but a necessity for busy moms. By prioritizing their own well-being, moms can better meet the needs of their families, maintain a sense of balance and fulfillment, and thrive in all aspects of life.

4

A Brief Background on Intermittent Fasting and Common Misconceptions

A. Intermittent fasting (IF) is an eating pattern that cycles between periods of eating and fasting. While it has gained popularity in recent years, intermittent fasting actually has roots that stretch back centuries, with practices of fasting being observed in various cultures and religions around the world.

One of the earliest recorded instances of fasting dates back to ancient Greece, where the philosopher Pythagoras advocated for abstaining from food for certain periods as a means of promoting physical and mental health. Fasting has also been a common practice in many religious traditions, including Christianity, Islam, Judaism, Hinduism, and Buddhism, often observed as a form of spiritual discipline or purification.

In the early 20th century, researchers began to explore the potential health benefits of fasting beyond its religious and cultural significance. In the 1930s, scientists discovered that calorie restriction—reducing calorie intake without malnutrition—could extend the lifespan of laboratory animals. This sparked interest in the effects of fasting on longevity and overall health.

Intermittent fasting gained further attention in the 20th century with the work of scientists such as Dr. Edward Dewey and Dr. Clive McCay, who conducted studies on intermittent fasting in animals and observed its potential benefits for health and longevity. However, it wasn't until more recent decades that intermittent fasting began to be studied extensively in humans.

In the 21st century, intermittent fasting has emerged as a popular dietary approach for weight loss, metabolic health, and overall well-being. Researchers have conducted numerous studies investigating the effects of intermittent fasting on various health markers, including insulin sensitivity, blood sugar levels, cholesterol levels, and inflammation.

Today, intermittent fasting has evolved into several different protocols, with popular variations including the 16/8 method (fasting for 16 hours and eating within an 8-hour window), the 5:2 method (eating normally for five days and restricting calorie intake for two non-consecutive days), and the alternate-day fasting method (alternating between fasting days and non-fasting days).

B. Debunking common myths and misconceptions about fasting

Despite its growing popularity, intermittent fasting is often surrounded by myths and misconceptions. Let's debunk some of the most common ones:

- Fasting leads to muscle loss: While prolonged fasting without adequate protein intake may lead to muscle loss, intermittent fasting, when combined with resistance training, can actually preserve muscle mass and promote fat loss.

- Fasting slows down metabolism: On the contrary, intermittent fasting has been shown to increase metabolic rate, particularly during fasting periods, as the body works to mobilize stored energy.

- Fasting is only for weight loss: While weight loss is a common goal of intermittent fasting, it offers numerous other health benefits beyond just shedding pounds, including improved metabolic health, cognitive function, and longevity.

C. Safety considerations and who should avoid intermittent fasting

While intermittent fasting can be safe and beneficial for many individuals, it's not suitable for everyone. Here are some safety considerations and groups who should approach fasting with caution or avoid it altogether:

- Pregnant or breastfeeding women: Fasting during pregnancy or while breastfeeding can deprive the body of essential nutrients needed for fetal development or milk production.

- Individuals with a history of eating disorders: Fasting may exacerbate disordered eating patterns or trigger unhealthy behaviors in individuals with a history of eating disorders.

- People with certain medical conditions: Individuals with diabetes, hypoglycemia, or other metabolic disorders should consult with a healthcare professional before attempting intermittent fasting, as it may affect blood sugar levels and require adjustments to medication dosages.

While intermittent fasting may not be suitable for everyone, particularly those with certain medical conditions or dietary restrictions, research suggests that it can be a safe and effective tool for promoting weight loss, improving metabolic health, and potentially extending lifespan. As interest in intermittent fasting continues to grow, scientists are continuing to explore its mechanisms of action and its potential applications for promoting health and longevity.

5

Understanding Intermittent Fasting

A. What is intermittent fasting?

Intermittent fasting (IF) is like a superhero strategy for busy moms looking to reclaim their health and energy levels amidst the chaos of everyday life. Instead of focusing on restrictive diets or complicated meal plans, intermittent fasting simply changes the timing of when you eat.

Here's the lowdown: Intermittent fasting involves cycling between periods of eating and fasting. But don't worry, it's not about starving yourself or going without food for days on end. Instead, it's about creating a schedule that works for you and your lifestyle.

One popular method is the 16/8 method, where you fast for 16 hours and eat during an 8-hour window. For example, you might start eating at noon and finish your last meal by 8:00 pm, then fast until noon the next day. During the fasting period, you can still drink water, tea, or coffee (without cream or sugar) to help keep you hydrated and curb hunger.

Another approach is the 5:2 method, where you eat normally for five days of the week and then limit calorie intake to around 500-600 calories on two non-consecutive days. These fasting days might sound intimidating, but remember, they're just a small part of your week, and you can still enjoy regular meals on the other days.

Intermittent fasting isn't about depriving yourself or feeling hungry all the time. In fact, many moms find that it simplifies their day and gives them more freedom with their food choices. By narrowing down the window of time when you eat, you naturally tend to consume fewer calories without even trying.

But the best part? Intermittent fasting isn't just about weight loss— it also comes with a whole host of health benefits. From improved insulin sensitivity and blood sugar control to increased energy levels and mental clarity, intermittent fasting can help busy moms feel their best and tackle whatever life throws their way.

So if you're a busy mom looking to boost your health and vitality without adding extra stress to your plate, give intermittent fasting a try. With a bit of planning and flexibility, you can harness the power of IF to reclaim your health and feel like the superhero mom you truly are!

B. The science behind intermittent fasting:

Let's break down the science behind intermittent fasting (IF) in a way that's easy to understand and apply to your busy lives.

Intermittent fasting isn't just another fad diet—it's backed by science and has some pretty cool effects on your body. Here's what's going on behind the scenes:

1. Fat Burning Machine: When you fast, your body doesn't have a fresh supply of food to burn for energy, so it starts tapping into your fat stores instead. This means you're essentially turning your body into a fat-burning machine, which can help with weight loss

and shedding those stubborn pounds.

2. Insulin Sensitivity: Ever heard of insulin? It's a hormone that helps regulate your blood sugar levels. When you fast, your insulin sensitivity improves, meaning your body can use insulin more effectively to shuttle glucose (sugar) into your cells for energy. This is super important for keeping your blood sugar levels stable and reducing your risk of type 2 diabetes.

3. Cellular Repair: Fasting triggers a process called autophagy, which is like a spring cleaning for your cells. During autophagy, your cells remove damaged components and recycle them into new, healthy ones. This helps keep your cells functioning optimally and can even slow down the aging process.

4. Hormonal Balance: Fasting can also have positive effects on your hormone levels. It increases the production of certain hormones like norepinephrine and human growth hormone, which can boost your metabolism and help preserve lean muscle mass. Plus, it can lower levels of insulin and inflammatory markers, which are associated with a host of health problems.

5. Brain Health: Believe it or not, intermittent fasting can also benefit your brain. Some studies suggest that fasting may improve brain function, increase the production of brain-derived neurotrophic factor (BDNF) which supports the growth of new neurons, and even protect against neurodegenerative diseases like Alzheimer's.

Now, I know what you're thinking—how the heck am I supposed to fit fasting into my crazy schedule? The good news is, intermittent fasting is super flexible and can be customized to suit your lifestyle. You can choose the fasting method that works best for you, whether it's fasting for a certain number of hours each day, a couple of days a week, or even just occasionally.

My favorite eating window is between 8:00 in the morning until 2:00

in the afternoon. That gives me an 18 hour fasting window. That might sound crazy, no food after 2:00 in the afternoon–"I'd starve!" But it works for me. My body has gotten used to it. I'm rarely hungry in the evenings anymore. If I do start getting hungry, it's late and I should be going to bed anyways. Just play around with the eating and fasting windows and figure out what your favorite is. You can always adjust or switch it around. That's the joy and ease of intermittent fasting!

So if you're looking to boost your energy levels, shed some extra pounds, and reap all the awesome health benefits that intermittent fasting has to offer, give it a try! With a little bit of planning and a whole lot of determination, you can harness the power of IF to become the healthiest, happiest version of yourself. You've got this, mama!

C. Why Intermittent Fasting is Easier Than Fad Diets

Intermittent fasting stands out from fad diets in several key ways, making it a more sustainable and practical approach for busy moms:

1. Simplicity: Unlike fad diets that often require complex meal plans, calorie counting (ugh!), and strict food restrictions, intermittent fasting simplifies the eating process by focusing primarily on when you eat rather than what you eat. This simplicity makes it easier to stick with long-term, as there's less mental energy spent on planning meals and tracking macros.
2. Flexibility: Intermittent fasting offers flexibility in terms of meal timing, allowing you to choose a fasting schedule that works best for your lifestyle. Whether you prefer to fast for 16 hours each day, restrict calories on certain days of the week, or alternate between fasting and non-fasting days, there's a method of intermittent fasting that can be tailored to fit your schedule and preferences.
3. No Food Restrictions: Unlike many fad diets that eliminate entire

food groups or demonize specific foods, intermittent fasting doesn't impose strict food restrictions. Instead, it allows you to eat a balanced diet that includes all your favorite foods, making it more sustainable and enjoyable in the long run.

4. Adaptability: Intermittent fasting is highly adaptable and can be easily integrated into your existing routine. Whether you're a busy mom juggling work, childcare, and household responsibilities, intermittent fasting can be adjusted to fit your schedule and lifestyle, rather than requiring you to overhaul your entire routine.

5. Focus on Health, Not Just Weight Loss: While weight loss is a common goal of intermittent fasting, its benefits extend beyond just shedding pounds. Intermittent fasting has been associated with improved metabolic health, increased energy levels, better cognitive function, and reduced inflammation, among other benefits. This focus on overall health and well-being aligns with the priorities of many busy moms who want to feel their best and stay healthy for their families.

6. Less Time-Consuming: Intermittent fasting typically requires less time and effort than traditional diets, as there's no need to spend hours planning meals, cooking elaborate recipes, or tracking every calorie. Instead, intermittent fasting allows you to simplify your eating routine and spend less time worrying about food, freeing up valuable time for other priorities.

Overall, intermittent fasting offers busy moms a practical, sustainable, and flexible approach to managing their weight and improving their health. By focusing on when you eat rather than what you eat, intermittent fasting can fit seamlessly into your busy lifestyle, making it easier to achieve your health and fitness goals without sacrificing precious time and energy.

6

How to Incorporate Intermittent Fasting Into a Busy Mom's Schedule

Incorporating intermittent fasting (IF) into an already busy schedule as a mom might seem challenging at first, but with some strategic planning and flexibility, it can be done. Here's a step-by-step guide on how to seamlessly integrate intermittent fasting into your routine:

1. Choose Your Fasting Window: Start by selecting a fasting window that aligns with your daily schedule and preferences. The most common method is the 16/8 approach, where you fast for 16 hours and eat during an 8-hour window. Consider your typical waking hours, meal times, and family routines when determining your fasting window.
2. Start Gradually: If you're new to intermittent fasting, consider easing into it gradually to allow your body to adjust. Start with a shorter fasting window, such as 12 hours, and gradually increase it over time as you become more comfortable with the fasting process.
3. Plan Your Meals: Once you've chosen your fasting window, plan

your meals accordingly. Depending on your schedule, you may prefer to skip breakfast and start eating around midday, or you may opt to have an early dinner and finish eating by early evening. Experiment with different meal timing strategies to find what works best for you.

4. Stay Hydrated: During the fasting period, it's important to stay hydrated by drinking plenty of water, herbal tea, or other non-caloric beverages. Keeping hydrated can help curb hunger and keep your energy levels up throughout the fasting period.

5. Listen to Your Body: Pay attention to your body's hunger cues and adjust your fasting window accordingly. If you find that you're feeling excessively hungry or fatigued during the fasting period, consider shortening your fasting window or breaking your fast earlier. It's essential to prioritize your health and well-being above sticking to a rigid fasting schedule.

6. Be Flexible: Understand that there will be days when your fasting schedule may need to be adjusted due to family obligations, social events, or other unforeseen circumstances. Be flexible and willing to adapt your fasting routine as needed to accommodate your busy schedule and lifestyle.

7. Stay Busy: Keep yourself occupied during the fasting period to help distract yourself from feelings of hunger. Engage in activities that you enjoy and that keep your mind off food, such as spending time with your children, tackling household chores, going for a walk, or practicing mindfulness and relaxation techniques.

8. Practice Self-Care: Finally, remember to prioritize self-care during the fasting period. Get plenty of rest, manage stress levels, and nourish your body with nutrient-dense meals during the eating window. Taking care of yourself is essential for maintaining your overall health and well-being, especially as a busy mom juggling multiple responsibilities.

By following these tips and making intermittent fasting work for your busy schedule, you can reap the numerous health benefits of IF while still managing your family and household duties effectively. Remember to listen to your body, stay flexible, and prioritize your health and well-being above all else.

7

The Power of Exercise for Busy Moms

A. Benefits of exercise for moms:

Now let's talk about exercise. Before you tell me there's no way, I don't have time or energy for that, let me just break down some of the amazing benefits of exercise and why you need it in your life.

1. Increased Energy Levels: It may seem counterintuitive, but expending energy through exercise can actually boost your overall energy levels. Regular physical activity helps improve circulation and oxygen flow, providing a natural energy boost that can help you power through busy days with ease. And don't we mamas all need more energy? Yes. Yes, we do.

2. Improved Mood and Mental Health: Exercise has been shown to release endorphins, which are chemicals in your brain that act as natural mood lifters. Engaging in regular physical activity can help reduce feelings of stress, anxiety, and depression, leaving you feeling more positive and resilient in the face of life's challenges. Every day is a challenge as a mom. Let's tackle these challenges

with improved moods and better mental health.

3. Better Sleep Quality: Quality sleep is essential for overall health and well-being, but it can be elusive for many busy moms. Regular exercise can help regulate your sleep-wake cycle, making it easier to fall asleep at night and enjoy deeper, more restorative sleep. Doesn't that sound wonderful?

4. Increased Strength and Stamina: As a mom, you're constantly on the go, whether you're chasing after little ones, carrying groceries, or juggling multiple tasks at once. Regular exercise, particularly strength training and cardiovascular activities, can help build muscle strength and endurance, making it easier to handle the physical demands of daily life.

5. Weight Management: Exercise is a key component of any weight loss or weight maintenance plan. By burning calories and building lean muscle mass, regular physical activity can help you achieve and maintain a healthy weight, which is important for reducing the risk of chronic diseases such as heart disease, diabetes, and certain cancers.

6. Improved Brain Health and Cognitive Function: Research has shown that exercise has a positive impact on brain health and cognitive function. Regular physical activity can help improve memory, concentration, and mental clarity, making it easier to stay focused and productive throughout the day.

7. Stress Relief and Relaxation: Exercise provides a healthy outlet for stress and tension, allowing you to release pent-up energy and unwind both physically and mentally. Whether it's a brisk walk outdoors, a yoga session, or a dance class, finding activities that you enjoy can help you de-stress and recharge. This benefit is number one for me! Taking care of four children all day long really takes it's toll on my stress/tension levels. Exercise is a wonderful outlet for me and makes me a much nicer person. If I go too many

days without getting to exercise, the whole family starts feeling the repercussions.

8. Social Connection and Support: Exercise can be a great way to connect with others and build a support network. Whether you join a fitness class, start a walking group with friends, or simply involve your family in outdoor activities, exercising together can strengthen bonds and provide a sense of camaraderie and encouragement. One of my most favorite things to do is to go on a walk or hike with family or a close friend. It makes for the best outing. Physical health and social health all wrapped up together.

In conclusion, exercise offers a multitude of benefits for busy moms, from increased energy levels and improved mood to better sleep quality and enhanced physical strength. By prioritizing regular physical activity, you can boost your overall health and well-being, making it easier to navigate the demands of motherhood with grace and resilience.

B. Finding time for exercise and incorporating it into your routine:

Finding time for exercise as a busy mom may seem challenging, but with some strategic planning and flexibility, it's entirely achievable. Here's a practical guide on how to find time for exercise and seamlessly incorporate it into your routine:

1. Schedule it in: Start by assessing your daily schedule and identifying pockets of time that could be dedicated to exercise. Treat exercise like any other important appointment and schedule it into your calendar. Whether it's early in the morning before the kids wake up, during nap time, during your lunch break, or in the evening after they've gone to bed, there are likely windows of opportunity that you can leverage for physical activity. Blocking

off dedicated time for exercise can help ensure that it doesn't get overlooked or pushed aside.

2. Prioritize Exercise: Treat exercise as a non-negotiable part of your day, just like any other important task. Block off dedicated time for exercise in your calendar and treat it with the same level of importance as other commitments. Remember, taking care of your health is essential for both you and your family.

3. Choose Efficient Workouts: When time is limited, focus on exercises that deliver maximum results in minimal time. High-intensity interval training (HIIT) workouts, circuit training, and bodyweight exercises are all excellent options for busy moms short on time. These workouts can be completed in as little as 20-30 minutes and provide a full-body workout.

4. Get creative and combine it with other activities: Look for opportunities to incorporate exercise into your daily routine. For example, you could take the stairs instead of the elevator, walk or bike to run errands instead of driving, do squats while brushing your teeth, or squats or lunges while you're cooking dinner, or calf raises while washing dishes. Every little bit of movement adds up!

5. Multitask Strategically: Look for opportunities to multitask while you exercise. For example, you could listen to an audiobook or podcast while going for a walk or run, catch up on emails or phone calls while using the stationary bike or elliptical machine, or do stretching exercises while watching your kids play at the park.

6. Involve the Kids: Don't be afraid to get the kids involved in your workouts. Turn exercise into a fun family activity by going for bike rides, playing active games like tag or soccer, or doing kid-friendly workout videos together at home. Not only does this allow you to spend quality time with your children, but it also sets a positive example of health and fitness.

7. Be Flexible: Understand that there will be days when your exercise

plans don't go as expected, and that's okay. Be flexible and willing to adapt your routine based on your changing schedule and circumstances. If you miss a workout, don't dwell on it—simply move on and make an effort to get back on track the next day.

8. Find Accountability and Support: Enlist the support of friends, family members, or online communities to help hold you accountable and stay motivated. Whether it's joining a workout group, finding a workout buddy, or tracking your progress in a fitness app, having support can make all the difference.

9. Make It Enjoyable: Choose activities that you genuinely enjoy and look forward to. Whether it's dancing, hiking, swimming, or practicing yoga, finding activities that bring you joy and fulfillment will make it easier to stick with them long-term. Remember, exercise doesn't have to be a chore—it can be something you actually look forward to!

10. Set Realistic Goals: Be realistic about what you can achieve given your current circumstances. Instead of aiming for lengthy workouts every day, focus on shorter, more manageable sessions that you can realistically fit into your schedule.

11. Celebrate Your Successes: Finally, celebrate your victories, no matter how small they may seem. Whether it's completing a workout, reaching a new fitness milestone, or simply making exercise a consistent part of your routine, give yourself credit for your efforts and progress.

By following these tips and making exercise a priority in your daily routine, you can find time to stay active and take care of your physical and mental well-being, even amidst the demands of motherhood. Remember, every little bit of movement counts, so don't underestimate the power of even short bursts of activity throughout the day. Embrace the opportunities to incorporate exercise into your busy life and reap the countless benefits it has to offer.

8

The Synergy of Exercise and Intermittent Fasting

When combined, intermittent fasting and exercise can amplify each other's benefits, creating a powerful synergy that promotes overall health and well-being. Exercise enhances the metabolic effects of fasting, while fasting may increase the body's ability to burn fat during exercise. Together, they form a potent duo that can help you achieve your health and fitness goals.

1. Enhanced Fat Burning: When you exercise in a fasted state, your body's insulin levels are low, allowing it to more readily access stored fat for fuel. This can enhance fat burning and promote weight loss, making exercise during fasting periods especially effective for those looking to shed excess pounds.

2. Improved Metabolic Health: Both exercise and intermittent fasting have been shown to improve metabolic health markers such as insulin sensitivity, blood sugar levels, and cholesterol levels. When combined, they can have a synergistic effect, potentially enhancing these benefits and promoting overall metabolic health.

3. Increased Energy Levels: Contrary to common belief, exercise

during fasting periods can actually increase energy levels rather than deplete them. This is because fasting enhances the body's ability to mobilize and utilize stored energy, providing a steady source of fuel for your workouts.

4. Optimized Performance: Some research suggests that exercising in a fasted state may enhance performance by promoting the body's ability to use fat as a primary fuel source. While more studies are needed in this area, many athletes and fitness enthusiasts report feeling more focused, energized, and mentally sharp during fasted workouts.

5. Appetite Regulation: Intermittent fasting has been shown to regulate appetite hormones, leading to decreased feelings of hunger and more controlled eating patterns. By exercising during fasting periods, you may further suppress appetite and reduce the likelihood of overeating later in the day.

Practical Tips for Busy Moms:

- Choose Convenient Workouts: Opt for workouts that fit seamlessly into your schedule and lifestyle. This could be a quick HIIT session at home, a brisk walk with the stroller, or a yoga routine during nap time.
- Stay Hydrated: Drink plenty of water before, during, and after your workouts to stay hydrated and support your body's performance and recovery.
- Listen to Your Body: Pay attention to how your body responds to exercise and fasting, and adjust your routine accordingly. If you feel overly fatigued or lightheaded, it may be a sign that you need to eat or rest.
- Be Consistent: Consistency is key when it comes to reaping the benefits of exercise and intermittent fasting. Aim to incorporate

both practices into your routine regularly, even if it's just for a few minutes each day.

By understanding the synergy between exercise and intermittent fasting and implementing practical strategies into your busy mom lifestyle, you can optimize your health, boost your energy levels, and achieve your wellness goals more efficiently.

As we conclude this chapter, I invite you to reflect on your own journey as a busy mom and consider how integrating intermittent fasting and exercise can enhance your life. Remember, self-care isn't a luxury reserved for those with ample free time; it's a necessity for all moms striving to be the best versions of themselves for their families. So remember to prioritize your health, embrace the journey, and celebrate the small victories along the way.

9

Real-Life Success Stories: Moms Who Have Embraced Intermittent Fasting and Exercise

To illustrate the real-world application of intermittent fasting for busy moms, we'll explore the stories of women who have successfully integrated fasting into their lives, sharing their experiences, challenges, and triumphs along the way.

1. Sarah's Story:

Sarah, a devoted stay-at-home mom, cherished her role as the primary caregiver for her three young children. From dawn till dusk, her days were a blur of diaper changes, school drop-offs, and endless household chores. Despite her unwavering dedication to her family, Sarah found herself neglecting her own health and well-being in the process.

Determined to make a change, Sarah turned to intermittent fasting and exercise as a means of reclaiming her vitality. Opting for the 5:2 method, she carefully selected her fasting days to coincide with her quieter moments at home. On these days, Sarah focused on nourishing her body with nutrient-dense meals, embracing the challenge of fasting with a sense of determination and purpose.

To incorporate exercise into her bustling routine, Sarah made the conscious decision to wake up early each morning for home workouts. Armed with nothing more than a yoga mat and a set of dumbbells, she transformed her living room into her personal fitness studio, carving out precious moments of self-care before her children awoke.

On weekends, Sarah seized the opportunity to escape the confines of her home and immerse herself in nature. Venturing out into the nearby wilderness, she embarked on long hikes through winding trails and towering forests, relishing the freedom and serenity that nature provided.

Through her unwavering commitment to intermittent fasting and exercise, Sarah experienced a profound transformation. She shed pounds, gained strength, and rediscovered a sense of vitality and purpose that had long eluded her. Her journey inspired those around her, serving as a powerful reminder that with dedication and perseverance, even the busiest of moms can prioritize their health and well-being amidst the chaos of motherhood.

2. Emily's Story:

Emily, a single mother of two young children and a busy corporate executive, faced the daily challenge of balancing her career with the demands of parenthood. Despite her hectic schedule, Emily was determined to prioritize her health and well-being.

To incorporate intermittent fasting into her routine, Emily embraced the 16/8 method. She decided to skip breakfast and delay her first meal until midday, allowing her to fast for 16 hours and eat within an 8-hour window. This approach not only simplified her mornings but also helped her reap the benefits of intermittent fasting, such as increased energy and mental clarity.

When it came to exercise, Emily got creative with finding ways to stay active without adding extra stress to her schedule. Instead of traditional workouts, she incorporated movement into her daily activities. For example, she would take brisk walks during her lunch break, do bodyweight exercises while playing with her children at home, and practice yoga or stretching before bed.

On weekends, Emily made fitness a family affair by organizing outdoor activities like hiking, biking, or playing sports with her kids. These activities not only allowed her to stay active but also provided quality bonding time with her family.

Despite the challenges of juggling work and parenting, Emily's commitment to her health paid off. She found herself with more energy, focus, and resilience to navigate the demands of her busy life. Emily's story served as an inspiration to other working moms, showing them that with a bit of creativity and determination, it's possible to prioritize health and well-being amidst a hectic schedule.

10

Strategies for Managing Hunger and Cravings

Managing hunger and cravings while intermittent fasting and keeping exercise in your routine can be challenging, especially for busy moms juggling multiple responsibilities. Here are some strategies to help you navigate these obstacles:

1. Stay Hydrated: Often, feelings of hunger can be mistaken for dehydration. Drink plenty of water throughout the day, especially during fasting periods and before and after exercise. Herbal teas, flavored sparkling water, and electrolyte-enhanced drinks can also help keep you hydrated and curb hunger pangs.

2. Fill Up on Fiber and Protein: During your eating window, focus on consuming filling and nutrient-dense foods that are high in fiber and protein. These nutrients help keep you feeling satisfied for longer and can help reduce cravings. Incorporate plenty of fruits, vegetables, legumes, lean meats, poultry, fish, eggs, and dairy products into your meals and snacks.

3. Choose Nutrient-Dense Foods: Opt for nutrient-dense foods that provide sustained energy and satiety, rather than empty calories

that can leave you feeling hungry and unsatisfied. Choose whole grains, healthy fats, and complex carbohydrates over refined and processed foods. Nutrient-dense snacks like nuts, seeds, Greek yogurt, and fruit can help curb cravings between meals.

4. Plan Balanced Meals: Plan and prepare balanced meals in advance to ensure that you have nutritious options readily available during your eating window. Batch cook meals and snacks that are easy to grab and go, such as salads, soups, stir-fries, and smoothies. Having healthy options on hand can help prevent impulsive eating and unhealthy food choices.

5. Practice Mindful Eating: Pay attention to your body's hunger and fullness cues and practice mindful eating during your eating window. Eat slowly, savor each bite, and stop when you're satisfied, rather than waiting until you're uncomfortably full. Avoid distractions like television or scrolling on your phone while eating, as this can lead to overeating.

6. Use Hunger-Fighting Strategies: If you experience hunger during fasting periods, try using hunger-fighting strategies to help manage cravings. Drinking black coffee or tea (without added sugar or cream) and distracting yourself with activities like going for a walk, reading, or engaging in a hobby can help take your mind off food.

7. Adjust Your Fasting Window: If you find that your fasting window is causing excessive hunger or cravings, consider adjusting the timing or duration of your fast. Experiment with different fasting protocols, such as shortening your fasting window, extending your eating window, or incorporating fasting on alternate days, to find what works best for your body and lifestyle.

By implementing these strategies and listening to your body's cues, you can effectively manage hunger and cravings while intermittent fasting and keeping exercise in your routine as a busy mom. Remember to prioritize nutrient-dense foods, stay hydrated, practice mindful eating, and adjust your fasting window as needed to support your health and well-being.

11

Creating a Supportive Environment at Home and in the Workplace and Staying Social

Creating a supportive environment at home and in the workplace while implementing intermittent fasting and exercise into a busy mom's schedule is crucial for long-term success. Here's a detailed guide on how to achieve this balance:

1. Communicate Your Goals:

Initiate a family meeting to discuss your health and fitness goals. Share why intermittent fasting and exercise are important to you, emphasizing how they contribute to your overall well-being and ability to be present for your family. Encourage open dialogue and ask for their support and understanding as you navigate these changes.

At work, consider scheduling a meeting with your supervisor or HR representative to discuss your wellness goals. Explain how intermittent fasting and exercise enhance your productivity, focus, and overall job satisfaction. Request any accommodations or adjustments to your schedule that would facilitate your ability to prioritize health during work hours.

2. Involve Your Family:

Get creative with ways to involve your family in your health journey. Set aside time for family meal planning and grocery shopping, allowing everyone to contribute their favorite healthy recipes and food choices. Schedule regular family fitness activities such as walks, bike rides, or backyard games to promote bonding time while staying active.

Empower your children by involving them in meal preparation and teaching them about the importance of balanced nutrition and regular exercise. Consider organizing family challenges or competitions to make fitness fun and engaging for everyone.

3. Set Boundaries:

Establish clear boundaries around your fasting and exercise routines to ensure they are respected by those around you. Communicate your schedule and commitments with your family, friends, and colleagues, and kindly decline invitations or requests that conflict with your health priorities.

Set specific times for your workouts and fasting periods, and communicate them to your family and coworkers. Encourage them to support you by respecting these boundaries and refraining from scheduling activities or meetings during these times.

4. Plan Social Activities Strategically:

When planning social gatherings, consider scheduling them during your eating window or at times that won't interfere with your exercise routine. Choose activities that align with your health goals, such as hiking, group fitness classes, or healthy potluck dinners.

Communicate your dietary preferences and fasting schedule with friends and family to ensure they can accommodate your needs when planning meals or outings. Offer to host gatherings at your home and prepare fasting-friendly dishes that everyone can enjoy.

5. Advocate for Yourself in the Workplace:

Take proactive steps to advocate for your health and well-being in the workplace. Research any wellness initiatives or programs offered by your employer and inquire about opportunities for flexible work hours, on-site fitness facilities, or wellness incentives.

Schedule a meeting with your supervisor to discuss your health goals and explore potential accommodations or adjustments to your work schedule that would support your intermittent fasting and exercise routine. Highlight the positive impact these changes will have on your productivity, focus, and overall job satisfaction.

6. Be Flexible and Forgiving:

Recognize that maintaining a healthy lifestyle while managing the demands of family, work, and social commitments can be challenging. Be flexible with your fasting and exercise routines, allowing for adjustments when necessary to accommodate unexpected events or changes in your schedule.

Practice self-compassion and forgiveness when faced with setbacks or deviations from your plan. Remember that progress is not always linear, and small setbacks are a natural part of the journey. Focus on making consistent, sustainable changes over time rather than striving for perfection.

7. Cultivate a Supportive Network:

Surround yourself with a supportive network of friends, family, and coworkers who share similar health and wellness goals. Seek out like-minded individuals in your community or online who can provide encouragement, motivation, and accountability as you work towards your goals.

Consider joining local fitness groups, online forums, or social media communities focused on intermittent fasting and exercise to connect with others who are on a similar journey. Share your experiences, challenges, and successes with your support network, and offer support and encouragement to others in return.

By implementing these detailed strategies and fostering a supportive environment at home and in the workplace, you can successfully integrate intermittent fasting and exercise into your busy schedule as a mom while still maintaining social connections and prioritizing your health and well-being. Remember that consistency, communication, and self-care are key to long-term success on your health journey.

12

Empowering Busy Moms to Thrive

As we reach the conclusion of "Healthy & Fit Moms: A guide for busy moms on losing weight and getting back in shape after babies," we reflect on the transformative journey we've embarked on together. Throughout this book, we've explored the intersection of intermittent fasting, exercise, and self-care, offering practical strategies and insights tailored specifically for busy moms striving to prioritize their health and well-being amidst the demands of motherhood.

1. Recap of Key Points

Let's take a moment to recap the key points covered in this book:

- Understanding Intermittent Fasting: We delved into the various methods of intermittent fasting, its metabolic and hormonal effects, and debunked common myths and misconceptions surrounding this dietary approach.

- The Benefits of Intermittent Fasting: From weight loss and improved metabolic health to cognitive benefits and longevity, we explored the myriad ways intermittent fasting can positively impact busy moms' lives.

- Why Intermittent Fasting is Easier Than Fad Diets: We discussed the flexibility, simplicity, and psychological benefits of intermittent fasting, showcasing testimonials of busy moms who have successfully transitioned from fad diets to a more sustainable approach.

- Incorporating Intermittent Fasting into a Busy Mom's Schedule: We provided practical tips for navigating the challenges of time constraints and juggling multiple responsibilities, offering strategies for meal planning, managing hunger and cravings, and creating a supportive environment at home and in the workplace.

- The Synergy of Exercise and Intermittent Fasting for Busy Moms: We explored the powerful relationship between exercise and intermittent fasting, highlighting the benefits of physical activity for energy levels, stress reduction, and mood enhancement, and providing strategies for integrating exercise into busy schedules.
2. Encouragement and Motivation for Busy Moms to Prioritize Self-Care

As busy moms, it's easy to put our own needs on the back burner while prioritizing the needs of our families and careers. However, it's essential to remember that self-care is not selfish but necessary for our overall well-being and ability to care for others.

- You Are Worthy: Remember that you are worthy of love, care, and attention, just like those you care for. Prioritizing self-care isn't a luxury but a necessity for maintaining your physical, mental, and emotional health.

- Small Steps Matter: Self-care doesn't have to be elaborate or time-consuming. Even small acts of self-kindness, such as taking a few moments to breathe deeply, going for a short walk, or enjoying a cup of tea, can make a significant difference in how you feel.

- You're Not Alone: Remember that you're not alone on this journey. Reach out to other moms for support, seek guidance from health professionals, and lean on your support network for encouragement and motivation along the way.

3. Final Thoughts and Resources for Further Support

As you continue your journey towards health and wellness as a busy mom, remember that progress, not perfection, is key. Celebrate your successes, no matter how small, and be gentle with yourself during setbacks.

- Resources for Further Support: Explore additional resources on intermittent fasting, exercise, and self-care to deepen your understanding and support your journey. Whether it's books, podcasts, online communities, or professional guidance, there are many avenues for further support and education.

- Your Journey, Your Pace: Remember that your journey towards health and wellness is unique to you. Embrace the process, honor your body's needs, and trust in your ability to navigate the challenges that arise along the way.

13

Some Extra Resources for You

Here are some resources that busy moms can use to learn more about implementing intermittent fasting and exercise into their busy schedules:

Books:

- "The Complete Guide to Fasting" by Dr. Jason Fung and Jimmy Moore: Provides comprehensive information on the benefits of fasting and practical guidance on how to incorporate intermittent fasting into your lifestyle.
- "Delay, Don't Deny: Living an Intermittent Fasting Lifestyle" by Gin Stephens: Offers a personal and relatable perspective on intermittent fasting, with tips for busy individuals looking to simplify their approach to fasting.

Websites and Online Communities:

- Reddit Intermittent Fasting Community (r/intermittentfasting): A supportive online community where individuals share their experiences, success stories, and tips for incorporating intermittent fasting into their lives.

- The Obesity Code website (https://www.obesitycode.com/): Features articles, podcasts, and resources by Dr. Jason Fung, a leading expert on intermittent fasting and metabolic health.
- Facebook Groups: There are many intermittent fasting Facebook groups where people share their success stories that are both relatable and inspiring. Information is also always being shared, so it's a great place to learn even more about intermittent fasting and all its benefits.

Apps:

- Zero: A fasting tracker app that allows users to track their fasting hours, set goals, and access educational resources and support from the Zero community.
- MyFitnessPal: A comprehensive app for tracking food intake, exercise, and weight loss goals. It can be useful for monitoring calorie intake and nutritional balance during eating windows.

Podcasts:

- The Intermittent Fasting Podcast by Melanie Avalon and Gin Stephens: Offers insights, tips, and interviews with experts on intermittent fasting, making it an informative resource for busy moms looking to learn more about the fasting lifestyle.
- The Fasting Method Podcast by Megan Ramos and Dr. Jason Fung: Explores various aspects of intermittent fasting, including its benefits for weight loss, metabolic health, and overall well-being.

Fitness Programs and Online Workouts:

- Beachbody On Demand: Offers a variety of fitness programs, including high-intensity interval training (HIIT), yoga, dance, and strength training, that can be streamed from home on-demand.
- Daily Burn: Provides live and on-demand workouts led by certified trainers, with options for all fitness levels and preferences.
- YouTube: There are so many free workout videos on YouTube that you can do right in the comfort of your living room. Just type in the kind of workout you're looking for in the search bar and take your pick.

Local Fitness Groups and Classes:

- Check out local gyms, community centers, or recreation departments for group fitness classes that fit your schedule and interests. Many facilities offer childcare services, making it easier for busy moms to attend classes.
- Look for outdoor fitness groups or mom-and-baby workout classes in your area, which provide opportunities to exercise while bonding with your little one and connecting with other moms.

Nutritional Guidance:

- Consider consulting with a registered dietitian or nutritionist who specializes in intermittent fasting and women's health. They can provide personalized guidance and meal planning strategies to support your fasting goals while ensuring adequate nutrition for you and your family.

By utilizing these resources, busy moms can gain knowledge, find support, and discover practical strategies for incorporating intermittent fasting and exercise into their busy schedules. Remember to listen to your body, stay flexible, and prioritize self-care as you embark on your health and wellness journey.

14

Final Wishes

As we conclude our journey together, I want to express my heartfelt gratitude for allowing me to be a part of your wellness journey as a busy mom. Thank you for choosing "Healthy & Fit Moms: A guide for busy moms on losing weight and getting back in shape after babies" as your companion on your journey. I sincerely hope that the book has provided you with valuable insights, practical tips, and inspiration to prioritize your health and well-being amidst the demands of motherhood. Remember that you are capable, resilient, and deserving of a life filled with health, happiness, and fulfillment. May you continue to prioritize self-care, embrace the power of intermittent fasting and exercise, and thrive in every aspect of your busy mom life.

If you found "Healthy & Fit Moms" helpful and empowering, I would be deeply grateful if you could take a moment to share your thoughts and experiences with others by leaving a review on Amazon. Your feedback is invaluable not only to me but also to other busy moms who may be seeking guidance and support on their own wellness journey.

Please consider sharing what resonated with you most about the book, whether it's the practical strategies for integrating intermittent fasting and exercise into your busy schedule, the inspiring success stories of fellow moms, or the encouragement to prioritize self-care and embrace imperfection.

Your review will not only help other readers make informed decisions about whether "Healthy & Fit Moms" is right for them but also serve as a source of encouragement and motivation for me to continue providing valuable content that empowers busy moms to thrive in every aspect of their lives.

Thank you once again for your support and for being part of the "Healthy & Fit Moms" community. I truly appreciate your feedback and look forward to hearing about your wellness journey.

Wishing you health, joy, and abundance on your journey ahead.

Katie Pruitt